My Path to Me

My Path to Me

Uniting Spirituality, Love, and Personal Development Through Discovering The Relationship With Myself.

Abel Calderon, Jr., Esq.

ISBN: 978-0-578-43244-1

Dedication

This book is dedicated to my son,
Abel Andres Calderon.

Son, know that when I felt most alone, loving you was the one thing I felt was true and authentic for me; and it was through the continued practice of loving you that I found my way back to loving me, loving God, and loving everyone and all things around me. Your life made the biggest difference in my life. With lots of love. - Dad

Special Acknowledgement

I now take the time to offer a special acknowledgement to all the teams who have supported me. My Sacramento St. Francis Catholic prayer group, SF8, PHD8, LP144, LP137, the Dream Connections Mastermind group, my family, friends, co-workers, attorney colleagues, and all who supported me through the process of writing and publishing this book. In particular, I thank Mr. Andrew Grace (Instagram: @andrewgracephoto and @andrewgracemusic) for his support with the cover photo and the audiobook, to Ryan Biore at 99designs.com for his support with the book cover design, and to Nikki Van De Car at KN Literary Arts, Lizette Balsdon at www.editingqueen.co.za and Rachel Cox on Fiverr for their support with the editing and formatting of the initial copies of this book.

Table Of Contents

Introduction

Some say it is impossible to reconcile the concept of "spirituality" and "personal development." However, I along with many others are already living the balance between the two. This book will support both ends of the spiritual and personal development spectrum (from those who cannot find the balance to those already living it), as well as everyone in between. The focus of this book is to explore what I believe to be the core of all religion and human experience: **spirituality**.

Spirituality, to me, is the very real and fundamental aspect of our existence — our non-physical, non-tangible self. If we are truly honest with ourselves, we must admit that there is a part of our human self that is not physical. Philosophers and scholars have referred to this part of us as "soul" or "spirit." For the purposes of our discussion, I will refer to this aspect of our human existence as spirituality—that ability in us to experience life beyond our five physical senses.

For me, spirituality transcends religion. This statement is not intended to be either a positive or negative statement towards any religion – it's entirely neutral, just as if I were to say that "emotions transcend the one feeling of love." In this book, I will convey discussions and experiences that are in no way intended to assert that any one religion is or is not better than any other religion, dogma, or creed. Instead, the purpose this book is to illustrate how, regardless of any creed or race, we are all similar in more ways than we give ourselves permission to acknowledge. Whether we want to admit it or not, we are all connected and traveling on the same path of personal discovery and enlightenment. Our individual moments differ, but collectively, our life experience is much the same.

The challenge of this book is that it is, in a way, a conversation on a topic that is beyond our human vocabulary and comprehension. For instance, some readers may have reservations around the use of the word 'God'. I respect and concede that not all readers may be in agreement as to whether there is a 'supreme being', but when I speak of God, I refer to that 'something' that connects us all together through spirituality – our non-physical nature and the source of it.

The fundamental premise of this book is that all human beings can experience non-physical realities; and our emotions are but one example. In fact, I propose that our ability to experience the non-physical is integral to whom we are as human beings, and that this ability is part of a greater consciousness, a consciousness which connects us all. I, therefore, refer to this greater and collective consciousness as "God," the source of our spiritual selves.

To illustrate this, I will share my journey, and how my perception of spirituality has evolved and expanded my awareness of myself and the world around me. I will explain how the discovery of my own spirituality rejuvenated many areas and aspects of my life that were stagnant and dormant. By uniting both personal growth and spirituality, I have reached levels of love, connection, joy, and peace that I did not know were possible. My wish for each person reading this book is that they will leave this dialogue with me with the ability to also create heightened levels in their own lives and to transcend any limitations regarding love, connection, and understanding of their own life journey. What is available on the other side will blow your mind and heart...I promise!

CHAPTER ONE:

Spirituality, A Relationship with Myself

If spirituality is my ability to experience the nonphysical; then—to truly understand 'my' ability—my discovery journey should at some point lead me back to 'me'. Although this may seem obvious upon first reading, my experience is that this is not always self-evident in practice. My spiritual journey as a child led me all over the place—everywhere, in fact, except back to 'me'."

I am of Mexican descent and grew up in a traditional Catholic family with traditional Latin values. This meant that authority was supreme, whether that authority was God or my parents. As a child, there was very little dialogue about any concepts that were uncomfortable, such as religion, sex, or politics. Instead, my experience of learning was to simply follow the rules and do what I was told was right and proper.

I still consider myself Catholic; in my journey of spiritual growth I have discovered great value in

Catholicism. But I will confess that seeing beyond the rules and the structure of Catholicism was not always easy as a child. Doing what we were told was crucial to our family, and if the rules were broken, we would be reprimanded or punished. Religion for me was the same: if I broke the rules, I was told that God would punish me. And if my sisters and I were good children, there would be a reward. When we did well in school or completed our chores, my mom would reward us. In the same way, I believed God would reward me for following the commandments and praying my prayers.

As a child, I felt that spirituality could only exist in the structure of religion. I believed that spirituality could only be practiced when reaching out to God. In other words, I believed that my spiritual ability had no purpose or function unless it was being used in the context of some "religious" act or event, such as prayer or Mass. I also felt that it was only through religion that I could discover more about this aspect of myself that I recognized was as real as speaking or hearing, my spirituality.

Although I appreciated the security of the structure of certain prayers, as I became older, the structure felt restrictive. There were times when I simply wanted to have a conversation with God, but when I would engage in these conversations with

God and experienced my spiritual ability transcending my religious upbringing, I felt as though I was doing something wrong; that it was a secret I could not tell anyone because somehow, this method was "improper"—even though it felt more natural to me.

Of course, all of this was simply my experience, and it is certainly not the case for every practicing Catholic. I hold no resentment towards Catholicism or my parents, and simply acknowledge that this is how I felt while trying to figure out the spiritual ability that I knew I had.

During college at St. John's Seminary College in Camarillo, California, I double majored in Spanish and philosophy and obtained a minor in psychology with an emphasis in theology. It was at the seminary that I realized that my impulse to converse with God was actually healthy and natural. I learned about Greek and modern philosophy and how men and women throughout history have attempted to understand spirituality, emotions, and the body as part of the entire human experience. I learned that to have questions and explore this aspect of myself was natural, normal, and a sign of maturity—not "wrong" as I believed as a child.

After college and throughout the last twenty years, I have read many books on personal growth, relationships, spiritual awareness, forgiveness, goal-setting, and positive thinking. I have also attended various workshops on emotional intelligence and relationships, as well as retreats on spirituality and self-awareness. As a result of all these experiences, I created and facilitated my own workshop on spirituality and the impact it can have on all relationships. Each of these has provided a unique perspective and clarity on what spirituality means to me and how it is central to my being.

Personal development has been the piece of my life puzzle that brought me this clarity. Through personal development I have obtained the clarity and the ability to acknowledge the aspects of me that are unique and valuable. I have discovered not only that these aspects of me are valuable but also why I must choose to "see" the value and what I am doing—or not doing—that is holding me back from embracing the value of the gifts that are innately part of who I am.

The greatest gift personal growth and self-awareness have given me is the concept of practicing "self-love". For as much as I prayed, or read scripture telling me that God loved me or that I was God's gift to the world, I never felt the true depth of love until I experienced my ability to offer *my* love to myself.

The challenge of self-love is to simply offer the same affection and enthusiasm that we would naturally give to someone else, and to it give ourselves at same level. The task is not complicated. We are called to continue to be the same loving, caring, thoughtful person we are to others, but to also include ourselves on the list of people who deserve the love we are willing to give to others. Although the concept made sense in theory, for me self-love was a very difficult concept to implement and to feel comfortable doing. I literally had to work at and practice being as loving and kind to myself in my acts and in my self-talk as I would be towards the first love of my life on our first date.

Personal development provided me one of the most profound realizations of my spiritual journey - to know and embrace that my own self-love is enough. For many years, I felt that to feel whole, complete, and adequate, I needed something external, something outside of myself, to provide me with…something – love, praise, affection, or acknowledgment. I have discovered that the "something" I was seeking outside me was the treasure within me.

Often, I would pray for God to "fill my cup" when I felt empty. I depended on the love of my family and friends to feel worthy and important. I engaged in acts or bought things or did what I considered "acts of kindness" in exchange for the affection that I felt I needed to feel that I mattered. Because I would use my acts and gestures of kindness as a currency for love, the experience became a transaction rather than a true act of love or sincere expression of affection. And I was using prayer in a similar way—only speaking to God when I needed something.

In addition to feeling that I was not enough, I compounded my lack of self-worth by engaging in negative self-talk. The most difficult habit to overcome was my negative self-talk. I would tell myself I was "stupid," an "idiot" or "less than" whenever I made an error in judgment, or whenever I did not receive the affection or the result I expected to make me feel important. When a relationship ended, I would tell myself "of course this happened to you; who would want to be with you?" And then I would look for reasons to justify the other person leaving me such as telling myself it was because of my physical appearance, my culture, my social status, or any other aspect of me that I did not like about myself. All these were examples of how I believed that I was not worthy and required "something" to "make" me worthy or loveable.

In my early twenties I experienced the joy of falling in love, and I recall the joy and excitement that flowed through my body and heart during that time. It was my first true love and through that relationship, my son was born. However, the relationship ended because of my lack of maturity during my early twenties. For many years, I carried the guilt and belief of being inadequate and unlovable, and I would use my own words to remind me of how I failed at the relationship.

I have since discovered that my greatest responsibility is the task of taking care of myself—not just my physical health but also my emotional and mental health. One of the most powerful ways to take care of myself is to be loving with the words I offer to myself. Using words of affirmation, compassion, and love toward ourselves should be as natural as breathing oxygen into our lungs. I believe that self-confidence is deeply rooted in how we speak to ourselves and whether we are willing to acknowledge the qualities and gifts we possess. I know that my inability to feel confidence was because I was holding myself low through the weight of my own words.

I discovered my love for myself is more powerful than any exterior love could be. This self-love is powerful and unique because it is endless! My ability to love me is sustainable. My ability to love me is a choice that is not only free but is available to me at any time. All I must do is choose to be loving, and do it.

My love for myself is AS powerful as God's love, and I stand 100% by this statement, because in truth, God's love and *my* love are one and the same. God's love flows through me and that same loving flow of power is the love I get to offer to myself. In my journey of spiritual growth, I have discovered that when I am unable or, more accurately, unwilling to love myself, I prevent the fullness of God's love or anyone else's love from entering my heart. To allow myself the ability to love me is a condition to receiving the fullness of anyone's love including the love of God.

To truly experience any kind of love, I must first let go of any limiting beliefs I might have. When I fully embraced that I am worthy and deserving of love, and therefore allowed the love of God and my loved ones to fill the limits of my heart, my life changed. From that moment, I was able to feel what it means to receive love in its pure and authentic form. To receive authentic and genuine love and affection is more valuable than any exchange for love I have ever experienced. And the love offered is unique and special because I am open to receiving it untainted by any reservations or expectations.

When I experience authentic love and affection because I am open to receiving it, I notice that I am not focused on the circumstances of the moment. Instead, the moment is authentic precisely because I am focused on the moment and not on the circumstances. What the person I am with is wearing, what I am wearing, how I look, how they look, their hair or clothing—none of these things matter in the moment of authentic love and connection. And in the same way, I am called to embrace me as I am, period, without judgement of my own circumstances or perceived limitations. This journey of spiritual growth through self-love should ultimately lead me to the complete acceptance of who I am.

To embrace and love every aspect of myself is the first step to taking my spirituality to the next level. Mind you, this does not mean I believe that I am perfect in every way. Rather, the goal, if you can say there is a goal, is to embrace myself in whatever moment I am in, no matter where I am in my journey, and to accept that this moment of my life is "perfect," or just as it is supposed be, because it is *my* moment in *this* particular moment.

Rather than judge myself for having chosen a path, or for being involved with a person, or not being where someone else is in life, or for having gone through a divorce, a betrayal, or any form of pain or heartbreak, I am called to embrace and love my journey and experience. This does not mean that I live a life of complacency, or that an emotionally difficult event was not a painful, or if I was abused that it was right. Rather, the intention is to embrace my experience as part of my own personal and unique journey. I am called to see and acknowledge that I overcame that moment, that I am greater, stronger, and more valuable than any circumstance or act of hate, and that, even when standing in front of the fire of the experience, *I choose* to love me because I matter and deserve to be offered the same love I would offer another.

Self-love opens limitless avenues for spiritual growth and healing. With complete self-love there is calm in my heart and peace in my body. In this space spirituality can be a healing ability to offer to myself first and then to others; self-love can be the most powerful healing agent if we allow ourselves the possibility of anointing our most difficult experience with the "sacred oil" of genuine self-love. With genuine self-love any internal wounds can heal.

My self-love can also inspire others, by being an example of how to be loving. Every person can offer their own gift of love to themselves. By loving myself, I can inspire those around me into their greatness, so that they can find the power within themselves to offer self-healing through self-love. And then, through our combined experience, we can take our individual abilities to higher levels, for each of us adds to the experiences of those around us.

Please note that the self-love I am describing is not a call to arrogance, egoism, or narcissism. Rather, it is a call to honor the self. It is a call to see our value and uniqueness, through loving ourselves. The difference between arrogance or ego, and the self-love I propose, is in the end purpose of the love. True self-love has the intention of honoring the self, with the purpose of acknowledging all that we are, to ultimately share this love through connection and unity with others. Ego and arrogance, on the other hand, inevitably involve separation and superiority, which does not lead to authentic connection or unity, but instead leads to isolation. True self-love is the honoring of myself so that I may see and honor the value in others.

I confess I was not always in this space of embracing my experience. Growing up, I felt I was expected to be "perfect." Unfortunately for me, I was a good student and obtained very good grades. This was unfortunate, not because education was bad, but because in my mind, I connected getting good grades with my mother's pride and joy for me. I believed that if I kept being the best in school, then my mom and family would continue to love me and that this love from my family meant that I was worthy and important.

To complicate my experience even more for myself, I attended a seminary to study to become a priest. For a Latino Catholic family, this was akin to sitting at God's table for dinner. My family, and my mom in particular, felt a strong sense of pride as I studied to be a priest and a servant of God. I believed that their pride in me meant that they loved me more. But after eight years of seminary education and only four years away from being ordained, I met a girl and fell in love.

I decided to take a break from the seminary and explore this experience of love, which was so profound, since it was truly my first love. I had dated in high school, but never felt anything this deep. This experience felt as though I was touching God through the touch of another. I felt in my heart and spirit that this love was a gift from God.

After dating for three months we began having sexual intercourse, which took the "love experience" to a higher level. I never realized what my body was capable of feeling when I combined love, emotional, and physical connection. To have my body feel in almost every cell the affection I held in my heart was transcendental. I felt as if I was able to turn my act of lovemaking into a sacred and religious experience of love.

This perception came crashing down when at twenty-two years old, straight out of the college seminary and without a job, we discovered she was pregnant with our son. My mom conveyed her heavy disappointment in me. I felt my family took me off the pedestal. Additionally, the priest mentors who I had great respect and honor for told me I was a disappointment. In my heart, I felt that because all these people who I loved were disappointed, God too must have stopped loving me. I eventually convinced myself that having sex and bringing a life into the world meant that my family and God stopped loving me, and so what I once thought was beautiful and sacred became dirty and a stigma.

My perception of myself, as being unworthy of love, made it very difficult to be open to anything but negative self-talk—the opposite of self-love. Although my ability to be spiritual did not leave me, I had very little desire to practice being connected to God when I felt so much unworthiness and self -

hate. The last thing I wanted to do was to speak to a God who I felt no longer loved me. So, I numbed my inner calling to be spiritual by turning to alcohol and cigarettes. I felt so much self-loathing that eventually it came out through my anger and hurtful words towards my partner and those around me.

My lack of self-love made it very difficult to allow joy in my life, indeed for anyone around me to be joyful or happy. Sadly, the person that I placed my hurt upon the most was the mother of my son. I expressed my hurt through words that demeaned and hurt her, and our relationship suffered tremendously because of it.

Prayer was not enough to "heal" me; it could not, because I was not in a place emotionally to allow that to happen. Emotionally, I simply did not believe I was connected to God. When I prayed, I simply recited words. It was no longer a conversation with God. I felt alone and believed that God was not listening.

I now know that during that time God was trying to speak to me and let me know God never stopped loving me. It was not that God was not speaking to me as much as that I was unwilling to admit that I was feeling hurt, angry and disappointed. The resistance to acknowledging my emotions prevented me from listening to God or anyone in my life. I was unwilling to listen because of the pain of my mom's words, the pain of words by my mentors, and the pain I felt from feeling judged by my family. I took that pain and blamed myself, and I couldn't forgive myself, much less love myself. My unwillingness to simply admit that I was feeling these emotions was the reason I could not hear God speak. I felt as though I was a failure, and the only way I knew how to handle this was to blame and emotionally beat myself up.

Ultimately, time allowed the hurt to subside, and as the hurt lessened, I was able to feel other feelings. My son became my miracle. Although I could not love myself, I could find in myself the ability to love him. With time I began to experience joy. The joy of being a father and playing trains with my son or feeling like a kid again every time my son and I watched cartoons or movies. This helped me experience other feelings. However, the underlying guilt was not addressed. It was simply ignored and suppressed.

I continued to avoid my feeling throughout my relationship with my son's mom. Rather than turn into the root of the self-judgement and guilt, I avoided the feelings and believed that if I simply focused on work, or played with my son, or stayed in the relationship out of obligation, that the guilt would take care of itself. As most have experienced, this approach rarely works. Instead, the guilt turned into unhappiness with myself, lack of self-love and a lackluster outlook on life. As my emotions manifested themselves in the relationship with the mother of my son, they took their toll causing the relationship to end; this became yet another emotional setback for me.

For thirteen years, I carried my guilt and sadness with me. Although I could not see it because I became accustomed to it, it was on my face and demeanor. I had no idea it was so obvious to everyone—I thought I had overcome it and "dealt with it." I had not. Instead, what I had really done was bury it. I took all my pain, emotions, hopes, and desires and placed them in a metal chest. I locked it up and buried it, never to be seen again. That is how I "handled" my pain.

After the divorce, I continued to avoid my guilt and hurt by isolating myself emotionally and devoting all my time and energy to law school and to my career as an attorney. I achieved great "success" which included passing the bar exam on the first try, having great results at trials, and becoming partner at my law firm, but did so at an emotional cost. I secluded myself in the process.

I believed that since I was successful at work, I had overcome my traumas. This was a complete misconception. If I was honest with myself, I would have noticed that most of my relationships had been sacrificed as a result and had become superficial. I did not have real, authentic connections with anyone. Only a handful of friends stuck around and that is more because of their love for me than my efforts in sustaining my relationships with them.

I don't know how long I would have gone on in that manner. I knew, on some level, I wasn't living an authentic, fulfilled life. As a result, I sought out books on self-awareness to find techniques on letting go of anger and tools on choosing what I wanted from life and finding happiness. However, I could not implement the concepts and tools in such a way that the results manifested in a way I could see them working. I stayed stuck in my head, thinking that if I understood the concepts intellectually or learned the techniques, this meant I had addressed my emotional baggage. Of course, understanding concepts and practicing techniques is only the very first step toward handling anything, but I was incapable of realizing that at the time.

Fortunately, I attended an emotional intelligence and transformational training event. This is where I finally was able to experience the concepts the books were attempting to explain. This is where I was exposed to what it meant to engage in the practice of loving myself rather than learning a technique. This is where the concept of "loving myself as much as I am willing to love others" landed. The concepts landed because I was invited to practice them and was partnered up with strangers who were committed to hold me accountable. These individuals chose to support me in my discovery because they had already experienced the training and desired simply to offer me the gift of self-love as their way of expressing their gratitude for their own discovery of self-love. No book I had previously read could do this for me.

As a result of these trainings at MITT in Los Angeles, owned by Margo Majdi; the Atlas Project in San Francisco with Dris Upitis; Mision Vital in Cerritos, California; The Fearless Man with Brian Begin and Dave Stultz; and through the years of practice with various amazing men and women, I reach new levels of awareness. Through the constant feedback on how I was showing up— whether I was being truly open and authentic or not – and the constant interaction and practice of vulnerability and sharing my experience, my emotions and my struggles, when I went back and read the same books on self-awareness, the depth of the messages of the authors, speakers, and mentors I had previously read or heard made so much more sense.

I am extremely grateful to all the authors, motivational speakers, public figures, and mentors who opened my mind and my heart to understanding that I deserved more: Napoleon Hill, Wayne W. Dyer, Louise Hays, Deepak Chopra, David DeAngelo, Zan Perrion, Marianne Williamson, Oprah Winfrey, Ellen Degeneres, Steve Harvey, Will Smith, Eckhart Tolle, Mark Edward Davis, Katherine Woodward Thomas, Dr. Robert A. Glover, David R. Hawkins, James Allen, Dan Millman, Don Piper, Viktor E. Frankel, David Dejda, George S. Clason, Paulo Coelho, Brendon Burchard, Gary Chapman, Dale Carnegie, Chandler Bolt, Lise Cartwright, Don Miguel Ruiz, Anthony Robbins, Zig Ziglar, Brian Tracy, Esther Hicks, Richard Carlson, Michael Alan Singer, Gabrielle Bernstein, Brené Brown, the Dalai Lama, Desmond Tutu, Armando Christian Pérez, Matthew Kelly, James C. Collins, Russ Harris, Dr. Joe Vitale, Russell Simmons, Elizabeth Gilbert, Warren Buffett, Lewis Howes, Josh Dodds, Sergio Lara, Patricia Ortiz, Nicole O'Brien, Rebecca Regnier, Lucero Rodriguez, Maryanna Ramos, Sandra Padilla, Torey Wolford, Lily Rose Marks, Ana Lídia Jiménez Colín, Sr. Guadalupe Muñoz, Lisa Foon, Michael Mabardy,

Brittany Murales, Gabriela Villacorta, Devon Luongo, Elaine Huang, Sergio Lopez, Michaela Yamamoto, Jorge Haddock, Michael Strasner, Chris Lee, Mary Joe Lorei, Krista Petty Raimer, Sylvia Badasci, and my parents: Maria Calderon and Abel Calderon, Sr., along with the writings and authors of Scripture, and many other individuals and sources who are all in my heart and too many to name here. Because of their words and works, I have been able to transform who I am emotionally, mentally, and spiritually.

As a result of these trainings, I began to discover how multi-faceted the concept of love is. Though I had always found ease in the concept of loving God, I never considered loving God as something that was optional. Having been raised in a Catholic family, in my mind, God was my creator and, therefore, I *had* to love God. I was perfectly fine with that deal. It was a way of showing my gratitude for my life.

Therefore, trying to apply the concept of loving myself as I loved God did not resonate with me. Although the idea of loving myself as I loved God seemed to be the logical and the easy next step, figuring out the ways to implement this concept seemed complex. The disconnect and confusion for me was that I did not know exactly *how* to love myself. I loved God, and demonstrated that love, by praying or going to church—but how was I to translate that into love for me? Was I supposed to pray to or for me, or spend quiet time for me?

I suppose those are fair options, but again, those felt foreign to me. I could not find the answer to the question until I asked myself the following: "Abel, how do you let people know that you love them?" I thought of course of my friends and family. I thought of how I buy them gifts or send a card or a message letting them know I was thinking of them. This, however, still did not resonate with me as feeling authentic. So, then I asked myself the following deeper question: "Abel, when was the last time you were wholeheartedly in love and how did you express your love during that time?" The answer to this question broke me. I realized I had spent the last thirteen years trying to forget that I had ever fallen in love. I had tried to live my life as if that event never took place in hopes that if I if I erased the memory of loving, then maybe the pain associated with the loss of the relationship could also somehow be erased from my heart and mind.

At first it was extremely uncomfortable to even remember what it felt like to be in love. I held so much resistance because I thought that if I remembered the love, I would inevitably remember the pain. But as I gave myself permission to remember how much in love I was with the mother of my son when I was dating her, I recalled the passion I felt, the excitement, how my body desired to hold her and how I also desired to be held and touched by her. I then noticed that I began to feel the creativity in my spirit become alive once again through allowing myself to feel these emotions and sensations in my heart and my body. I realized my heart was not broken or a damaged aspect of me; I simply had not allowed my heart or my body to feel.

I recalled how those emotions sparked in me the desire to write poems and drive for hours to simply spend thirty minutes with her. I recalled how much I loved my son and the joy of playing trains with him. I recalled how I worked two jobs to make sure I provided for them both to make ends meet while living in a converted garage. I recalled how I made sure my son had enough to eat even if it meant that I would not eat dinner that night.

It was only by going through this process of remembering, from the memory of my heart, that I was able to understand *how* I was supposed to show love to myself. I was being called to be enthusiastic about my achievements, and passionate about overcoming any struggles that might come my way in the same way I was passionate about seeing the girl that I loved and willing to do anything to be with her. I was called to apply this passion towards my goals and dreams. I was called to not only write but to daily speak poetic and loving words to myself and give myself words of encouragement when I felt alone or overwhelmed. I was called to be vigilant over my health and my wellbeing, in the same way that I was vigilant for the health and sustenance of my son and wife. Loving myself required treating myself as an equal, giving myself the *same* I was willing to give to others when I showed and expressed my love and affection. This concept changed my life!

At first, I didn't think I could do it. It felt awkward and unnatural, and I tried to convince myself that this was a dumb idea. My mind argued that even if I tried it, it would not change my "screw-ups" or mend the past. Thankfully, my heart was my neutral advocate that said, "just try it." I took a risk and chose to listen to my heart. I gave myself permission to let my heart lead this time. In the past, I only let my mind lead because I was not ready to trust the wisdom of my heart. However, all the books on personal development gave me the courage in that moment to be open and risk since in the end, I knew it was my heart who was asking me for my love. I chose to no longer deny my heart my own love.

My mind has been my protector, and I have grown to love and appreciate it. The mind is like that friend that tries to keep us safe even when it pushes us over into the ditch trying to protect us. And regardless, I love my mind. I believe that my mind has the genuine desire to keep me safe, although it may not exercise the best judgement. Moreover, my mind is still learning how be tactful in how it says and does things. If my mind has engaged in negative self-talk or self-criticism, it is because I have allowed my mind to speak to me this way and because I have allowed others to speak to me with way. My mind has simply been a student. Fortunately, I have learned to stand up for myself and quiet the negative self-talk my mind churns out. Relying on my heart and my spirit has supported me to balance the judgment of my mind. With their help, I have essentially given my protecting mind an early retirement.

Transitioning from self-criticism to self-love is largely dependent on being vigilant and rigorous in our language and on the level of commitment we choose to hold when speaking to and about ourselves. The words we speak and we how we speak them creates the world around us. To transform my world, I must first transform how I speak to and about me. **Transformation starts with our language.**

Although it may be our intention to be loving, if we do not change the language we use towards ourselves, then our love—like any other love to another—will not thrive. Negative self-talk and criticism are like the weeds in the garden that will eventually kill the roses. It is my responsibility to be vigilant that no weeds take root in the garden of my mind and heart through my negative self-talk.

Some may relate to their minds as I did with mine, and if you do, please understand that not everything your mind thinks or says through negative self-talk, is true. Again, your mind is simply attempting to protect you. For others, it may not be your mind, but your emotions that take you places that cause pain. I invite you to be loving to this aspect of yourself and acknowledge that emotions are a way of fulfilling your desire to connect and love. Using your spirituality, by connecting to your intuition and practicing being the neutral observer of your experience, may be the missing piece which helps you to find the balance of how to guide your emotions, so that through the spiritual guide, the emotions can lead you to the places and relationships that will be sustainable and positive.

Know that your emotions feel, while your intuition sees. Allow your intuition to guide you as you sort through the feelings. In the end, all are called to balance the information of our mind, with the desire of our emotions, through the wisdom of our intuition and inner insight. Spirituality is the playground where all these can come together and through their harmony provide us all we desire.

My mind was right: loving myself did not erase any of my painful experiences or any of my mistakes. But to erase the past is not the purpose of self-love. The purpose, if there is one, is that self-love will allow me the permission and ability to embrace my journey as a learning experience. My self-judgment and self-hate did not give me permission to make a mistake—how could I learn when I expected myself to be perfect? I expected myself to hit a homerun every time I went to bat.

I couldn't even acknowledge the deep love I had for my wife and my son because I believed that since the relationship ended, that meant the entire experience was worthless. I refused to recall that when I saw my wife for the first time, it was love at first sight. I fell head over heels for her! I refused to acknowledge how attracted I was to her, and that for me, she was the most beautiful and sexy girl I had ever seen. She was in my thoughts throughout the day, and every time I received a letter from her, my entire body felt joy and excitement.

After our relationship ended, my mind swept these emotions of love and joy under the proverbial rug and focused only on the pain and the events surrounding the hurt. My mind tried to keep me safe by remembering only the things that would justify my feelings of hurt—so that I wouldn't fall in love again, and possibly be hurt again. Self-love allowed me to see my entire love story and acknowledge that love did exist.

Similarly, for a long time, when I spoke of my mom's reaction to my having a child and becoming a dad, I only recalled the pain of my mom's disappointment. By acknowledging the pain and embracing this experience through self-love, I was able to be see that the pain was not the whole experience. I was able to acknowledge that my mom had many wonderful attributes as a mother: strong, loving, deeply rooted in her faith, committed to her children and family, and overwhelmingly generous with her time and resources. I was not being fair to my mom by holding her to one event, when she had been loving and giving in countless other moments both before and after the event – from the day I was born to, when I saw her last and made me dinner as

I visited her. Self-love allowed me to see her entire story, as well as my own.

Self-love helped me regain the ability to see my experience through other people's perspective. I was able to acknowledge that my mom was genuinely disappointed, and that in that moment she was experiencing many emotions and did not have the ability to express her disappointment in a way that would have been sensitive to how I was feeling. Although I may not agree with the way she handled it, taking the time to put myself in her position gave me the ability to understand why she reacted the way she did, and this provided additional healing for me.

And with my ex-wife, by learning to be loving towards my experience, I was able to acknowledge that my lack of love for myself took its toll on her, and that despite my hurtful behavior, she remained faithful to me and my son until we divorced. Taking responsibility for my role *while at the same time* embracing that I, at twenty-five years old, did the best I could in that painful situation, allowed me to see what I could learn to improve my future relationships. Yes, the lessons were tough and painful, but I can honestly say that now, because of practicing self -love for my experience, I would not change one bit of the pain I went through. It is part of the fabric of who I am today.

Because I am finally able to love myself, including loving all the "mistakes" and "errors" I made, I now find it so much easier to love and forgive others. I find it easier to feel and experience the love and affection of others. I can enter a conversation and quickly see the beauty and vulnerability of the person in front of me because I see it in myself. Most importantly, I have experienced the fullness of God's love because I have learned to love myself.

Before, I felt as if I was experiencing sunlight from the inside of a house through a little window. Now I feel like I am outside and feeling the sunlight touching and warming my entire body. I was unaware of how I limited my spiritual ability because I was not practicing self- love, and now I am beyond grateful at how much love I can experience, from all sources, as a result of this practice.

This ability to love myself has also impacted how I now treat my body, how I regulate my self-care, and how much kindness and love I offer the vessel that holds my spirit. Learning to practice self-love has naturally included loving and honoring my body. In the past I would criticize my body as being too short, or too fat, or not being attractive. I was also unkind to my body in other ways which included not giving my body enough sleep, eating unhealthy food, and over indulging in alcohol and drugs.

Self-love has helped me embrace me exactly as I am, to nurture my body, and to accept that my beauty is not necessarily in my physical appearance. I have embraced that my true beauty and honor lies in what I can do with the body I am given rather than what it looks like – how many heartfelt embraces can I give, how many words of encouragement can I offer, how many smiles can I provide. Acts of love are what people remember and desire from me more than my perceived imperfections. And to love and honor my body is how I can express gratitude to God for the gift of my body and how I can let others know I love them—I love them enough that I choose to care for me, so that I can continue to sustain my ability to engage in further acts of love and affection for the benefit of us both.

CHAPTER TWO:

Spirituality, A Relationship with Others

The next step in our journey of spiritual growth is to develop our relationships with others. For a long time, I believed that if I had a relationship with God or if I meditated or prayed, this proved I was spiritual. It was easy to tell myself, "Since I am connecting with God, this should be the same or better than connecting with others." My mind justified my "going to the source" as the best option to be connected to God, though it in no way required me to be in relationship with those around me. In fact, I was using spirituality to keep me from connecting with others.

I now know that my spiritual ability finds fullness when it connects and engages with the spirituality of others. Although connecting one-on-one with God is deeply powerful, coming together in community to share our struggles and our human experience with each other and offering each other love and support, takes our spiritual ability of connection to higher levels. Human connection through spirituality is one of the most unique and profound experiences available to us. It is one thing to experience God's love, but to experience God's love while connecting with the love and affection of the people around us takes the experience to a level that words cannot describe. We can experience God's physical touch through the touch and embrace of those around us.

Again, this was not always my experience of spirituality. Recall that my way of handling the pains and disappointments of my life was to isolate myself. Having a private relationship with God felt more natural to me, because this was how I believed I was to live my life – on my own and without depending on anyone.

My parents divorced when I was four years old, and as a child the experience taught me that disappointments should be handled by the individual, not the collective. I learned this from observing my mom and how I believed she handled her divorce. My mom rarely talked to us about the pain or loneliness she experienced. She handled her emotions by praying, going to Mass every day, and listening to songs about lost or impossible love relationships, which she would then enjoy singing to us. My interpretation was "don't talk about your emotions", "handle disappointments on your own", and "use prayer and spirituality and music to let out the pain". From this, I deduced that if I let God know what was going on in my life, God would heal the pain, and I would not need to let anyone else know what I was feeling.

This interpretation of the events in my early life naturally promoted isolation and encouraged not being in communication about my emotions. I felt that sharing any emotions that were not strictly positive would be a burden I was foisting on others. As a child, I never told my mom that I missed my dad because I saw how much sadness she was already experiencing, even though she would not tell us directly. I felt she was going through a difficult time and decided that I would not tell her how I was feeling, since I did not want to cause her more pain by sharing my own feelings of loneliness and sadness. In my mind I felt that if I shared my feeling, this would add to her own sadness and cause an additional burden upon her.

For high school and college, I attended a seminary to explore the vocation of becoming a priest. As part of my education, I studied western philosophy and experienced priests as being above normal men – independent males, always capable of overcoming the pull of emotions, especially the desires for sex and intimacy. Western philosophy generally depicts emotions as less valuable than the mind, logic, and reason. My interpretation of this was that my emotions were simply feelings with no benefit, and the sooner I got over them, the faster I could move on with my life and with achieving my goals which at that time centered on praying, studying and trying to be a devote "priest in training."

For me, practicing being a priest meant that I had to develop the ability to not feel any emotions or sexual desires; the sooner I learned this, the better it would be for me because as a priest, I would need this skill in my ministry to be an effective and devout servant of God. So, I practiced not being able to feel anything so that it would be easier to handle emotions when they did arise. Of course, not only was this a complete misconception of how to be an effective priest but trying not to feel any emotions was physically impossible.

Rather than it becoming easier, my attempt to avoid feeling any emotions became increasingly difficult and frustrating. Since I could not stop feeling emotions, I instead developed the mindset that emotions were to be treated as secret things that I might feel, but would pretend did not exist, so that I could continue to maintain the image of what a priest or an independent man was supposed to look and act like. Even after I left the seminary, I continued to practice this way of dealing with my emotions. I would be unwilling to share my struggles or communicate any of my emotions or situations that bothered me because I had convinced myself that emotions had no value.

As I learned about how to live a more balanced life, I knew that I needed to expand my perception of emotions. Though I tried to deny it, I was blessed that my heart had the ability to feel all emotions—not just the socially acceptable ones of joy and happiness—despite my pretending it could not. Personal development helped me to understand that emotions are essentially neutral feelings—happiness is not better or worse than anger, for instance. What matters is what I do with the feeling, and whether the actions I take lead me to what will serve me. The feelings themselves do not create anything, but the actions we take in response to our emotions create the outcome that either serves us or not. Ultimately, emotions—when observed and perceived from a neutral perspective—can be guides to understanding ourselves and what is unique to our personalities and our life journey.

This is not to say that emotions become easier to experience or are less intense. On the contrary, my emotions flow more fluidly through me because by not judging them, I am actually allowing them to pass through me as they should. Emotions are like a breeze or a storm that is there in the moment and then passes to allow another moment to occur and another emotion to be felt.

In the past, I would regularly judge my feelings of sadness or loneliness. I felt that because these were not joy, they were bad. I also judged them because I feared them. In my mind I was resistant to these emotions and believed that to feel them meant that I was not strong. For me strength was defined as the ability to never feel loneliness, fear, or sadness. My fear of pain and sadness was so strong, I was ready to do all I could to not feel them.

I have now discovered that emotions have never been my enemy. Instead, if I allowed them, they could be my teachers. For example, sadness and loneliness taught me about who I really am and what my heart desires. When I listen to them, these emotions confirm I am a living being that longs and desires for connection and physical affection. I am someone who wants to know I matter to another living being. These emotions remind me of the need to not only be willing to express my affection but also the need receive the affection of others. Sadness and loneliness have taught me to not fight them. If I allowed them to lead me rather than resist them, they could show me who I truly am—a loving and connected man who desires to love and be loved.

For a long time, I believed that I did not need to be told "I love you," and that I did not need to be embraced. I believed that since I had survived without having the love, emotional support, or the affection of my dad, I really did not need the affection of anyone. Once again, my mind was trying to keep me safe. In my mind, if I could overcome the need to feel loved, then I would not have to ever deal with the pain and disappointment of that love being taken away. But my mind failed to acknowledge that—even though I may not have had my dad's affection as a boy—I experienced affection from many sources throughout my life.

Through personal growth, I am now able to step back and see the truer and bigger picture beyond the simplistic "I am alive and do not need anyone" viewpoint. By being sincere and taking the time to see the truer picture, I realized that even though I did not have my dad's affection growing up, I had the affection of so many other people—my mom, my two sisters, uncles and aunts, cousins, teachers, mentors, and friends.

There have been so many men that God put into my life that have served as a father figures for me: Bill Simons, Msgr. Alfred Hernandez, Fr. Thomas Boudreau, Bishop Edward Clark, Bishop Arturo Lona Reyes, Fr. Francisco Vitela, Professor Mariano Lopez, Professor Roland Glover, Professor Richard Geraghty, Roberto Mendez Palau, Tio Luis Tapia, Tio Abuelo Jesus Viveros, Richard Goldman, Paul Magdalin, George Krikes and many other priests, professors, colleagues, family members and mentors throughout my life. I have also been blessed with many close male friends who I consider brothers: Thao Dinh, Sergio Lopez, Mike Ramos, Andrew Grace, Sergio Lara, Brian Pecha, Nick Brooks, Travis Ross, Ray Rappold, Daniel and Moises Vargas, Eddie Lee, Armando Lee, Patrick McGinn, Peter Komenksy, my cousins in Mexico and Parlier, and my brothers OLQA Seminary, St. John's Seminary, and transformation leadership brothers at MITT, Atlas, Fearless Man, and Dream Connections.

Despite all that support, in my heart I missed my dad so much—of course I did. But I thought that these feelings of sadness provided me no benefit, and would lead me to depression if I paid attention to them. I thank God for providing me with a healthy system of feelings. This sensitive heart I have is so healthy and working so well that as much as I attempted to suppress these feelings, the emotions kept rising to the surface like little bubbles to let me know, "Hey, there is something down here that you may want to address." Emotions have been the gentle reminder that further healing is required.

Ultimately, by embracing my emotions and listening to the wisdom they had to offer, I rebuilt the relationship with my dad. We had a conversation and expressed how much love we have for each other and have always had for each other while, at the same time, acknowledging my dad's absence during my childhood and the pain it caused me were valid experiences for me. Now, I have both the love of my dad and the relationship with him I always prayed to have. And as an added bonus, I also have the love and affection of all the spiritual dads and brothers I have created while searching for my connection with other men. My search has not only brought healing to me but has also brought healing to men who were also searching for their own connections to other men. Thank you emotions, and thank you God, for leading me even when I did not know where I was going!

Even more powerful than feeling emotions is the act of sharing them. By giving myself permission to speak of my pain, sadness, and loneliness, I opened my heart and expanded my ability to connect. To my surprise, speaking of what I feared most and thought no one cared about, gave others permission to speak about their own emotions and personal experience. By speaking of my struggles and listening to the struggles of others, I discovered that so many us feel the same way, and that many times we have been through similar experiences. It was only through the sharing of our experiences that we discovered how similar we are, creating true connection.

That said, opening your heart and sharing your experience, is a vulnerable activity. I invite everyone who will be expressing what is held in your heart to be prudent in how, where, and to whom you share, so that you can continue to feel safe in doing so. Sharing in spaces and under circumstances where there is honor, respect, and most importantly, confidentiality, will serve you as you openly share, so that you will not be in a situation where your truths will be revealed without your consent or before you are ready to have your experiences and life story out in the open. As you practice, you will eventually develop the confidence in yourselves to share and not be attached to any judgment or fear of the secrets or experiences being shared. But start by working in a safe, judgment-free space until you reach this point.

I believe that one of God's greatest gifts to me has been my ability to feel God's presence through my connection and interaction with another human being. To connect my spirit with the spirit of another through conversation, prayer, or touch, is to feel God's kiss and embrace upon my spirit. To have my body experience this connection while feeling the connection of our spirits is akin to experiencing heaven.

I believe spirituality finds its fullness when I allow my individual self to connect and become one with the collective of the human experience - to experience the "oneness" of all humanity and of all things. This oneness becomes possible only in the practice of sharing and connecting at the deepest level with those around us. I believe we are called to openly, authentically, and vulnerably share our human experience with each other: the joys, the sorrows, the celebrations, what we perceive as our disappointments, the painful moments, and the moments of rejoicing that we each live. We all experience circumstances and the emotions they generate, and it is only in sharing them that we create connection with each other. When I withhold my experience, I am essentially affirmatively choosing not to connect; and to choose isolation is to deny

myself the gift of human connection and God's
ability to embrace me through the arms of another.

CHAPTER THREE:

Spirituality, A Relationship with God

The third step on our journey of spiritual growth is explore and develop our relationship and connection with God. Our relationship and perception with God must be a living and changing experience because we are living and changing. Spirituality is a practice; it is not a destination or a thing to be mastered. I grow and become a clearer vessel to receive and pass on the gifts of spirituality through the constant connection and contact with the Divine.

God is the source of our spirituality and the source of our connecting ability. The divine fabric which makes up God is the same divine fabric that makes up our spirit, and this includes our ability to feel and express our emotions and love. All emotions flow through our spiritual self and are then felt by our being. It is our mind that attempts to interpret our emotions and many times reduces the emotions into concepts. Emotions are not meant to be conceptualized. They are meant to be felt through our spirit. Love without spiritual connection is like a body with no life running through it; it is something reduced to a gesture where it can be an expression of

47

something words can never capture. To discover our spiritual fullness and full capacity to love, we must connect with the source of it without any limitations.

In the past, my perception of God was a force that existed outside of me. I would regularly pray to God to answer a prayer or to help me take care of something. I certainly believed that God was superior to me and beyond my grasp—in fact, I had been taught that if I actually "saw" God, I would die.

As I have grown in spirituality, I now perceive God differently, though I still feel the utmost respect and awe. I no longer perceive a separation, but rather a connection with God. I believe that God, through my spiritual ability, has granted me the power and the right to be a co-creator.

In the same way the planets are all part of the universe, I feel as though I am a planet on the same orbital field as God—not less or more than, but rather connected through spirit to God. God is the universe, and I am a planet, and although objectively, we may seem different, the molecules and matter that make up the essence of the universe are the same molecules and matter that make up the planet. The essence is the same.

To understand the power within me, a being made of the same fabric of God, I am called to discover this power. The method of discovery lies in developing an actual relationship with God. Where before my prayers felt more like ordering something from a menu and hoping I would get it, I now find myself having conversations with God. I speak and God listens. Then I maintain silence to allow God to speak so that I may listen, and for me God speaks through my ideas and emotions.

As I develop my ability to understand God's language, I grow in my capacity to connect with all that God is and has available for me to experience. It is in this space of deep connection that I then offer my requests in the form of a prayer and know that God is listening. God and I become partners in the creative process of my hopes and dreams. My goals and dreams become natural manifestations of God's abundance and love for me, which I then get to share with the world—this book being one example of this manifestation.

I believe that the concept of attraction and spiritual manifestation are really one and the same energy. Under the principle of attraction, when we have our intention clear in our mind, "the universe will conspire to make it happen". For me, prayer and desiring the manifestation of the object of my prayer is no different from the concept of attraction; it's just that we use different words to explain the same energy. Under both concepts, there is a goal which we desire to manifest, and being completely clear and completely emotionally committed to what we want are the key ingredients to manifesting that desire. And of course, both require the declaration and an exchange of action to move the creation process to full physical manifestation in our lives.

My communication with God has the power to manifest miracles. When my desires are infused with strong emotion to create, unrelenting commitment, and the activity which is congruent with my feelings, desires, and my heart, these then call *all* the energy of the universe—which is God—to co-create with me to bring my heartfelt desire to fruition. So, whether it is attraction or a calling to God through my spiritual connection to the Devine and its answer to me, the process is the same.

Personally, I find empowerment in knowing that I am in relationship with God and that when I call with my heart and am willing to exchange my efforts for what I want, God, through the universe, will answer. To know that God is listening overwhelms me with joy and love. When I pray and God answers, it is as though God is embracing me and whispering in my ear: "Yes, I am here for you."

My greatest epiphany through growing my relationship with God has been the shift in my perception of what "faith" now means to me. As a child, I felt that faith meant simply believing in God, who I could not see, hear, or touch. To believe without seeing was "faith". Now faith means so much more. I believe that God desires for me to use the power of faith to also believe in my goals and dreams. My faith has the power to bridge time and space between me and my goals, between not actually seeing them now and, through faith, develop the courage to believe that all my desires and dreams are possible for me.

The practice of believing in God is no different from the practice of believing in myself or believing that I am worthy of obtaining my dreams and goals. To live spirituality is to put my faith to practical use. By using the power of faith to believe in something I desire but cannot see in the moment, is, for me, a way of honoring God's power and love for me. When I allow for spirituality to become the lens through which I see life, God becomes human and faith becomes the tangible vehicle I can use to transport me to my destination—my goals.

If it is possible to use faith to believe in God, then it is also possible for us to take that same power and practice of faith to believe in the value and possibility of our heart's desires and manifestation. I believe this is how God desires for us to use our faith—to believe in God, *and* to believe in all that is possible for us when we are connected with God. The power of faith is God's creative force within us, and to practice that faith to the fullest of its potential is our way of affirmatively allowing God the ability to use everything at God's disposal for our benefit.

A genuine relationship with God has provided me with the ability to acknowledge that I am one with God, that I am connected and made of the same fabric as God and that God openly and without limitations invites me to connect with God at any moment. It is my birth right to create, and I am called to use the power of my faith to empower me to use all my gifts to the best of my ability for the betterment of myself and others. Through the continued practice of this, my relationship with God will only continue to grow and expand, and I will continue to be a vessel of the Devine in human form as is everything else around me.

CHAPTER FOUR:

Spirituality, A Relationship with Everything

The last step on our journey of spiritual growth is to explore and embrace our connection to everything. For as co-creators, we are stewards of creation. Having a relationship and being connected with God implies I am bestowed with the responsibility to honor and to be in relationship with everything God has created. I believe we are all called to live this responsibility and privilege every day—and the journey begins and ends with each of us. As I acknowledge the value and honor in me, I will find it easier to see the value and honor in all that is around me. This practice will naturally bring me back to the oneness of all things, and it will become my ongoing responsibility to affirmatively choose to embody the oneness connection which can flow through me and through all that is around me, moment to moment.

My journey of spiritual growth initially attempted to find fullness outside of myself, but as I journeyed within, I discovered my own value. As I recognized my value, I was called to love all aspects of who I was, especially those aspects of myself which I viewed and judged as faults or inadequacies. Through this practice of self-love, I experienced the love of God and the love of others.

As I grew in love, I noticed that my capacity to love was greater than the body that appeared to contain it. I began to focus outward and discovered the value of human connection as opposed to the limited one-on-one relationship with God I thought was all I needed. The more I connected with those around me and embraced our collective human experience, acknowledging our similarities by feeling and experiencing true, authentic affection and love freely offered, the more I understood the depth and limitless power of God and God's love within me. I discovered that my love was God's power alive within me.

Through this love and connection to others, I have discovered that I am called to see God and myself in all things. I can co-create, consume, and be a steward; and when I consume, I must choose to do so in a way that honors the dignity of the Divine in what I am consuming or transforming from nature.

To live this way is to honor sustainability. Personal growth and spirituality call us to be stewards of creation by acknowledging the responsibility we have for all creation. Love requires nothing less.

If there is a desire in me to destroy or to take, I believe that this is an internal reflection of where I am in my journey of spiritual growth. I believe that any desire that does not honor creation, whether it is not honoring our body or not honoring an individual or any object of creation, is a manifestation of a deep internal and personal lack of self-love or self-value within the person. Whenever this happens, the invitation is to go back to chapter one and start once again with the practice of self-love; so that we may seek out the part in us that feels the need to fill a void or lack. For it is only by honoring creation that we maintain congruence with the energy of love, and it is only in the continued practice of self-love that we become master stewards of creation.

Knowing that I am connected to all things brings me a unique sense of peace and love for myself and for everything around me. Ultimately, this is the peace that I believe that we all seek – the calmness and certainty of knowing we are one, that there is no beginning or end, and that we are contributing as much to creation as the tree that provides oxygen for us to breathe or the breeze that passes through the feathers of the birds as they soar through the sky.

By implementing this model of spirituality into my life, the ownership of providing the safety for the tree to grow and flourish so that I and all creation can breathe, grow, and flourish naturally flows. It is not an obligation, but rather an expression of love. To be a steward of nature is simply one way to express authentic care and affection for all of God's creation, of which I am also a part. This is what spiritual connection is—oneness with all things.

If it is not your regular practice to be with and in nature, then I invite you to take up the challenge of implementing this activity into your spiritual practice. Give yourself permission to feel nature caress your hair and face, embrace your body with the warmth of the sunlight, and whisper to your heart through the wind and breeze. Let nature remind you that you and it are one in the same; that nature is here to take care of you and provide you with what you need in exchange for your willingness to protect it, and that even when you forget, nature will continue to provide until it can no longer do so. Give yourself permission to recognize this call from nature, and then choose how you will respond. And as you decide, know that this practice and your response to nature is available to you in every moment and with every breath you inhale and exhale.

CHAPTER FIVE:

One Outline for Prayer

Although spirituality is not physical in form, it is like a muscle that we can train by engaging in it through continuous practice. The more we explore and play with various aspects of spirituality, the wider our experience becomes; and therefore, the more powerful our ability to develop connection with ourselves, God, and all that is around us. Note that I use the word "play" intentionally. I do so because my desire is that this practice be a loving and—if possible – joy-filled practice, as a child plays with their favorite toy and playmate.

First, I invite the reader to practice with the tools that are most comfortable to him or her. If there are words or activities you are accustomed to using, then start with those. Once you have your comfortable structure or approach in place, the next step is to engage in whichever posture feels comfortable to you. This can be sitting down, or standing, or kneeling. You can also use a candle or other items to engage the senses.

And as you engage in your normal practice or prayer style, then add the following: give yourself permission to speak and feel the words from your heart. Whatever the words are, whether a prayer or a meditation chant, practice saying these from the heart and soul rather than simply speaking them from the mind.

Feel the emotion you want to convey in your prayer or meditation, and let your body also connect to that emotion. Let these emotions and unspoken words pass through you. Notice what happens as you let the emotions be felt, in your body and your heart, before you speak them. Once you have processed your emotions and woven them into your words, then offer them as you pray your emotional desires to God. To pray from a place of offering our words and emotions and desires to God will create new possibilities for connection through spirituality.

As you pray or meditate, remain a conscious observer of your mind and heart. Notice whether your mind is distracting you or whether you have created such a deep connection that your mind becomes an open container to receive. Is there resistance, or is there love and honor for the experience.

As you observe, practice offering love, compassion, and affection to yourself and your experience. Allow your prayer or meditation to be an act of love for you and for your connection to the Divine. If there is pain and sorrow or loneliness and grief, let those emotions flow through you, and give yourself permission to see the gifts in each of these feelings, the vulnerability in them, and then acknowledge that you are healthy for feeling them. Although you may need to express and share your hurt or sadness in your offering, the experience can still be within a loving, safe and honor-filled expression.

Whatever the cause of the emotion you feel, let it be; choosing not from right or wrong, but rather, from "this is my experience, this is what I am feeling in this moment, and I honor it". Then embrace the you that is currently connecting the Devine with your love, and truly accept and acknowledge the strength and valor it has taken for you to be where you are at this moment. There is beauty, honor, and grace in this moment if you give yourself permission to see it, experience it, and embrace it.

As we practice this daily, it will become more natural to be loving. At first, it may feel weird or awkward. This is normal. All things done for the first time feel awkward, like writing with your left hand if you are right-handed. My request is that you trust, and continue to practice the exercise daily until it feels more natural.

For some, this experience may bring up deep rooted emotions. Know that this is normal, and that the healing process is in our ability to forgive ourselves. I believe that when we experience a traumatic event, we need to find forgiveness before we can release our emotional ties to this trauma. I offer the following as one approach for inner forgiveness and healing. We must 1) forgive ourselves for whatever we feel we did or didn't do in the moment that caused the event; 2) We must forgive the person or people involved for what they did or failed to do that resulted in the event; 3) We must forgive life for creating the circumstances that placed us in that place and at that moment of the event; and 4) We must forgive God for allowing the event that occurred to happen to us.

This process may be difficult at times. It has taken me several years to reach the point where I feel true forgiveness at all four levels regarding my life traumas. Of course, remembering the events still cause me some sadness, but I am no longer angry or resentful. I can now have a conversation about an event, acknowledge that it was difficult, and embrace that I am a stronger and a more compassionate person because of the experience.

Ultimately, forgiveness is reaching a point where I can face my event or experience, acknowledge it, and disconnect the emotional ties that are holding me back from moving forward. Once this is complete, then the healing can occur. I can then take it upon myself to take the emotions tied to the event and convert that event into a celebration of myself — where I once felt abused, I can convert it to my being resilient and courageous for overcoming the event; where I once felt abandoned, I can convert it to me acknowledging my strength, determination, and honor in transcending the circumstance. Forgiveness is not only moving past the event, but it must also call us to celebrate our life for our journey of transcendence over the event.

Although I did not use psychotherapy or a psychologist, these professionals do provide great benefit, and I encourage the use of professionals to anyone who believes they would benefit from their guidance. I have greatly benefited from sharing with mentors and from confiding in people who would listen to me when I was struggling with forgiving myself and others for the experiences I endured.

Another way of praying is to choose a specific emotion and make that emotion the lens that filters the entire conversation, so that the emotion adds its flavor to the words. I regularly choose gratitude as my emotion of preference and pray in this particular sequence. You can choose whichever emotion you feel would serve to elevate your connection with God.

First, I start my prayer by feeling gratitude in my heart and in my body, and let the feelings of gratitude flow through me. With the feelings present in me, I convey to God and offer God my joy and gratitude for the gift that I am, gratitude for all that I bring to others, gratitude for where I am in this moment in my life, appreciation for my accomplishments and gratitude for the things I still have an opportunity to accomplish. By conversing with God in this way, I honor myself for the miracle that I am, embrace my value, and let God know that I see the gifts God has given me, and that I am grateful.

I continue by further thanking God for being part of my life, and for granting me the wisdom to practice connection and gratitude. I ask God to continue to bless me and keep me grounded in love and appreciation for myself and my relationship with God and others. I express my gratitude to God for all those around me, as well as my ability to grow in relationship with them, because I realize that this is also a way in which I can physically experience God's love.

In the same spirit of gratitude, I then convey my appreciation for the gift of specific people in my life. I make it a point to name the person, whether it is my son, mom, my sisters, or my dad, and allow the feeling of gratitude and love to fill my heart and body. I pray for them and their wellbeing, and that God continue to help them reach their goals and give them the strength and wisdom through their own faith to overcome any obstacles they may be experiencing. Throughout this experience, I allow my emotions to be connected to my words so that I speak from my feelings of gratitude. My words are not empty and I imagine that, as I am praying for these specific people with feelings of love and gratitude, they are receiving these emotions in their hearts, regardless of where they are in the world.

As I pray, I also make it a point to acknowledge in my heart what specifically each person has done for me, how each has made a difference in my life, and how I am a better person because of the gift of them. I also take the time to notice all the other people in my life who offer value: people at work, those who are part of my social groups, friends, and anyone else I value. I take the time to honor those around me so that I maintain the desire to continue to be in relationship with them, and ask that God bless them and help them in whatever it is they need.

Only after acknowledging my gratitude, do I convey my needs. From my heart and emotions, I have a conversation with God, and I let God know what I am going through, the struggles and feelings I am experiencing. I let God know my fears and my frustrations. I express my pain and let God know how much it hurts. In times when I am completely overwhelmed, I let God know that I feel this way, that I cannot see where I am supposed to go or what I am supposed to do, and yes, sometimes this does bring me to tears. I let whatever feelings I have flow.

It is because of my vulnerability that I find the courage to surrender myself to the wisdom of God and allow God to provide me the ways that best support me in addressing my situation and in ultimately accomplishing my goals. I convey from my heart what I want, and what drives me to accomplish what I want—my goals, dreams, and desires.

I offer all these to God so that God can bless me and my goals and so my faith can provide me with the courage, commitment, and fortitude to reach my goals. I believe with all my heart that all things are possible when my desires are aligned with my purpose in life and with God's master plan.

Although at time the details may not turn out the way I had imagined, God has always provided me with the essence of what I have asked. And many times, God's ways have exceeded anything I could have ever imagined.

Finally, I pray for the qualities and personality traits that I want to embody, so that the time between where I am now and where I want to be, is a journey of inspirational growth rather than a struggle to achieve. I usually pray for wisdom, humility, love, discipline, trust, faith, joy, love, being open to shifting my approach, and above all, remaining grounded in the truth that my value is greater than any goal or ideal I may have. Enjoying the journey is as important—if not more important—than getting to the destination; and, yes, I also pray for the faith to believe wholeheartedly in this statement, and the strength to be true to my faith.

Of course, there are times when I struggle, but knowing that God is a loving and compassionate God provides me with the safety of returning to my loving co-creator to strengthen me when I feel I cannot keep going any further. I also take it upon myself to reach out to friends and family to share my struggles. I do so not because they will provide me with an answer or solution but because I know that they are God, who is made manifest in them, listening to me and letting me know that I am never alone.

A moment of disappointment never means I am not worthy, or that I am incapable of achieving. Many times, all it means is that I simply get to reconnect with God, confirm my desire, and keep going, or perhaps attempt a new approach. If my heart in prayer continues to pull me towards my desire, then this is confirmation that I must persist, because my desire matters! Finding the balance between achieving my desires as I want them and what God has destined for me only occurs in spirituality and through the ongoing conversations and relationship with God and those around me.

As you practice these different prayer options or your own version of it, go back to this book and ask the following: What would it be like if today I committed to being the joy I want in the world? If today, I committed to being the love for others that I desire, and if today I am the open heart in the world to make this possible? Feel what that feels like, to know that you have that power to create this change, and that these opportunities are available to you at every moment. It truly is a choice. Each of us is God's co-creator!

Feel and imagine what would it be like if today, I chose to truly embrace my value and self-worth? What would it be like if today I chose to make a phone call to reach out to someone who I have not connected with—who would that be? What if I openly discussed my struggles and frustrations so that the other person felt safe to speak about what they are going through? What if when they spoke, I simply listened, providing a safe space so that they can truly feel heard, appreciated, and loved? What if I embraced that I can be God made manifest for others? In that space, I would not feel the impulse to provide any answers. Instead, I would simply convey love and appreciation for them because that is the most pure version of God in us. Know that this is what our loved ones want: our love, not our advice or judgment. All they want to hear is us saying, "Thank you for trusting me and know that I love you." This is God's message to us and the same message we are called to share to others.

What would it be like if my relationship with God reached such a level that it would allow me to see my connection with all things and all people? What would it be like if I committed to honoring the littlest plant, animal, or rock as if I could see the sacredness in them? Would it possible for me to see and feel that in doing so, I would be honoring the sacredness of my relationship with God and that in a very real way, I become God present in the world?

As you ponder these possibilities and questions, be in the gift of silence and practice letting God speak to you. Allow God to speak through your emotions, your thoughts, and your spirit. Let whatever comes up just come up. Write these things down, so that what comes up is remembered. Create urgency around any answers from God that call for a change. If God is speaking, we must listen and promptly act on what is spoken to us.

Now, take the time to ponder on this final reflection: how would my life transform if I lived this practice every day? What would be possible in my life? What if I shared my love and affection with one person today? What if I allowed my heart to connect with one other person or an element of nature today and allowed my spirit to connect to the spirit of another and with the spirit of nature? What if I listened through my heart and spirit to the person or thing in front of me in addition to listening with my ears? What if I made these practices part of my regular way of life?

This is what is available to each of us at any moment. And as you let this last statement resonate with your heart and spirit, in *this* moment, I embrace you, connect with you and whisper to your soul, "this level of connection *is* possible in every area of your life if you choose it". The gateway is self-love, and the process is the practice of nurturing the mind and heart through the spirit. There are thousands of practices available to assist you growing and developing your connecting ability, including books and events that will inspire you to continue the journey of personal growth and intimate connection by remaining attuned to your emotions, your heart, your body, and your mind. Remember that your spirituality has the power to harmonize all aspects of yourself. By connecting to Source, you connect to the true you and it is only through the lens of love that you will have the ability to see and experience your greatness.

I pray that your life will be filled with abundant and authentic connections and that one day, we will connect in person and embrace.

The End

About the Author

Abel Calderon, Jr. was born and raised in Los Angeles, California. He attended Queen of Angels High School Seminary in San Fernando, California, St. John's Seminary College in Camarillo, California and then attended Southwestern School of Law in Los Angeles. He has participated and coached in various workshops on leadership, emotional intelligence, and spiritual awareness. He created his own emotional intelligence workshop focused on spirituality and relationships while in Los Angeles. He currently provides coaching while maintaining his role as a senior attorney managing the Central and Northern California practice at MacDonald, Ebbing & Lloyd, LLP in a Sacramento, California, which specializes in Workers' Compensation law for the defense. Mr. Calderon values and adores his family, his relationships with people from all walks of life, and the journey of self-awareness. His desire is for everyone to discover their own path to creating love, joy, and awareness though spirituality and connection, and that this book will provide a guide as each person embarks in their own unique and the incredible journey of discovery.